HEALTHY LIVING AND NATURAL LIFE PROTECTION

BY
AILEEN R. SCOTT

Copyright © 2023 by Aileen R. Scott

All rights reserved.

Table of Contents

Eat balance diet 8

For grown-ups 9

For babies and small kids.. 11

Down to earth guidance on keeping a sound eating routine 12

Leafy foods 12

Fats 13

Salt, sodium and potassium 14

Sugars 16

advancing sound weight control plans..................... 17

Consume less salt and sugar.. 22

Limit salt consumption 25

Limit sugar consumption 27

Lessen consumption of harmful fats 29

Eating less fat.. 31

Eliminating soaked fat 32

At the shops... 32

At home 33

Eating out 35

Keep away from unsafe utilization of liquor 38

Factors influencing liquor utilization and liquor related harm39

Be active 43

Good reasons to be more active 43

Being active Doesn't Need to Be Hard 44

Be active with Family and Make New Companions 45

Remain active so You'll be Free as You Age 46

The significance of being actually active outside 47

Youngsters 48

Grown-ups 48

Check your blood pressure consistently 50

requirements to screen circulatory strain at home 51

Kinds of home screens 53

Elements to consider.. 54

Gadget precision 55

Tips for precise use.. 55

Following your circulatory strain readings........................... 58

Long-term benefits.. 59

Practice safe sex 61

Unprotected sex might jeopardize you of STIs 61

Sorts of condoms... 63

Instructions to utilize condoms effectively 66

Different tips for more secure sex 67

Other more secure sexual practices.............................. 69

Keeping away from dangerous circumstances...................... 70

Conquering boundaries to safe sex...................................... 70

What to do on the off chance that you suspect a few side effects of STI
.... 72

Converse with somebody you trust assuming you're feeling down   75

Side effects and examples.. 77

Contributing variables and counteraction 79

Diagnosis and treatment.. 80

Drink safe water 82

Water and wellbeing 84

   Financial and social impacts 87

   Challenges.. 88

Take anti-toxins just as recommended 90

   Extent of the issue 91

   Counteraction and control 93

   People.. 93

   Strategy producers 94

   Wellbeing experts.. 95

   Medical services industry 96

   Agriculture area... 96

   Late turns of events... 97

   Influence 97

Introduction

Great nourishment, day to day practice and satisfactory rest are the groundworks of sound living. A sound way of life keeps you fit, vigorous and at decreased risk for infection. Sound living is an approach to living that assists you with getting a charge out of additional parts of your life. An approach to everyday life brings down the gamble of being truly sick or biting the dust early. Wellbeing isn't just about staying away from a sickness or disease. It is about physical, mental and social prosperity as well.

At the point when you embrace a solid way of life, you give a more certain good example for others in your family, especially kids. You will likewise establish a superior climate for them to experience childhood in. By assisting them with following a better way of life, you will be adding to their prosperity and delight in life now and later on.

Overseeing pressure in sure ways, rather than through smoking or drinking liquor, lessens mileage on your body at the sub-atomic level. For a more extended and more agreeable life, you ought to embrace a solid way of life.

Chapter 1

Eat balance diet

Eat a mix of various food varieties, including natural product, vegetables, vegetables, nuts and entire grains. Grown-ups ought to eat no less than five parts (400g) of products of the soil each day. You can work on your admission of foods grown from the ground by continuously remembering veggies for your feast; eating new products of the soil as bites; eating different products of the soil; and eating them in season. By practicing good eating habits, you will decrease your gamble of hunger and non-transferable infections (NCDs) like diabetes, coronary illness, stroke and malignant growth.

Consuming a sound eating regimen all through the life-course assists with forestalling unhealthiness in the entirety of its structures as well as a scope of non-transferable sicknesses (NCDs) and conditions. Notwithstanding, expanded creation of handled food varieties, quick urbanization and changing ways of life have prompted a change in dietary examples. Individuals are currently devouring more food sources high in energy, fats, free sugars and salt/sodium, and many individuals don't eat enough organic product, vegetables and other dietary fiber like entire grains.

The specific make-up of a differentiated, adjusted and solid eating regimen will shift contingent upon individual qualities (for example age, orientation, way of life and level of active work), social setting, locally accessible food varieties and dietary traditions. Notwithstanding, the fundamental standards of what comprises a solid eating routine continue as before.

For grown-ups

A healthy diet include the following :

•Organic product, vegetables, legumes (for example lentils and beans), nuts and entire grains (for example natural maize, millet, oats, wheat and earthy colored rice).

•Somewhere around 400 g (for example five bits) of leafy foods each day (2), barring potatoes, yams, cassava and other bland roots.

•Under 10% of all out energy consumption from free sugars (2, 7), which is identical to 50 g (or around 12 level teaspoons) for an individual of sound body weight consuming around 2000 calories each day, however in a perfect world is under 5% of complete energy consumption for extra medical advantages (7). Free sugars are sugars added to food varieties or beverages by the producer, cook or shopper, as well as sugars normally present in honey, syrups, natural product squeezes and natural product juice condensed.

•Under 30% of absolute energy consumption from fats (1, 2, 3). Unsaturated fats (tracked down in fish, avocado and nuts, and in sunflower, soybean, canola and olive oils) are desirable over soaked fats (found in greasy meat, margarine, palm and coconut oil, cream, cheddar, ghee and fat) and trans-fats, all things considered, including both economically created trans-fats (tracked down in heated and broiled food sources, and pre-bundled bites and food varieties, like frozen pizza, pies, treats, rolls, wafers, and cooking oils and spreads) and ruminant trans-fats (tracked down in meat and dairy food varieties from ruminant creatures, like cows, sheep, goats and camels). It is recommended that the admission of soaked fats be decreased to under 10% of all out energy consumption and trans-fats to under 1% of all out energy admission (5). Specifically, economically delivered trans-fats are not piece of a solid eating regimen and ought to be kept away from (4, 6).

•Under 5 g of salt (identical to around one teaspoon) each day (8). Salt ought to be iodized.

For babies and small kids

In the initial 2 years of a kid's life, ideal sustenance cultivates solid development and works on mental turn of events. It additionally lessens the gamble of becoming overweight or large and creating NCDs sometime down the road.

Guidance on a solid eating routine for babies and youngsters is like that for grown-ups, yet the accompanying components are likewise significant:

- Newborn children ought to be breastfed constantly until 2 years Babies ought to be breastfed only during the initial a half year of old and then some.
- From a half year old enough, bosom milk ought to be supplemented with various satisfactory, protected and supplement thick food varieties. Salt and sugars ought not be added to corresponding food sources.

Down to earth guidance on keeping a sound eating routine

Leafy foods

Eating something like 400 g, or five parts, of products of the soil each day decreases the gamble of NCDs (2) and assists with guaranteeing a satisfactory day to day admission of dietary fiber.

Products of the soil admission can be improved by:

- continuously remembering vegetables for feasts;
- eating new foods grown from the ground vegetables as bites;
- eating new foods grown from the ground that are in season; and
- eating an assortment of leafy foods.

Fats

Diminishing how much absolute fat admission to under 30% of all out energy consumption assists with forestalling undesirable weight gain in the grown-up populace (1, 2, 3). Likewise, the gamble of creating NCDs is brought down by:

- decreasing immersed fats to under 10% of complete energy admission;
- diminishing trans-fats to under 1% of complete energy consumption; and
- supplanting both immersed fats and trans-fats with unsaturated fats (2, 3) - specifically, with polyunsaturated fats.

Fat admission, particularly immersed fat and mechanically delivered trans-fat admission, can be decreased by:

- steaming or bubbling as opposed to searing while cooking;
- supplanting margarine, grease and ghee with oils wealthy in polyunsaturated fats, like soybean, canola (rapeseed), corn, safflower and sunflower oils;
- eating diminished fat dairy food sources and lean meats, or cutting back apparent excess from meat; and
- restricting the utilization of heated and seared food sources, and pre-bundled tidbits and food sources (for example doughnuts, cakes, pies, treats, rolls and wafers) that contain mechanically delivered trans-fats.

Salt, sodium and potassium

The vast majority consume an excess of sodium through salt (relating to consuming a normal of 9-12 g of salt each day) and insufficient potassium (under 3.5 g). High sodium consumption and lacking potassium admission add to hypertension, which thus expands the gamble of coronary illness and stroke (8, 11).

Diminishing salt admission to the suggested degree of under 5 g each day could forestall 1.7 million passings every year (12).

Individuals are frequently uninformed about how much salt they consume. In numerous nations, most salt comes from handled food sources (for example prepared dinners; handled meats like bacon, ham and salami; cheddar; and pungent bites) or from food varieties devoured regularly in huge sums (for example bread). Salt is likewise added to food varieties during cooking (for example bouillon, stock solid shapes, soy sauce and fish sauce) or at the place of utilization (for example table salt).

<u>Salt admission can be diminished by</u>:

- restricting how much salt and high-sodium sauces (for example soy sauce, fish sauce and bouillon) while cooking and getting ready food varieties;
- not having salt or high-sodium sauces on the table;
- restricting the utilization of pungent bites; and
- picking items with lower sodium content.

Some food manufacturers are reformulating recipes to lessen the sodium content of their items, and individuals ought to be urged to check nourishment names to perceive how much sodium is in an item prior to buying or devouring it.

Potassium can moderate the adverse consequences of raised sodium utilization on pulse. Admission of potassium can be expanded by consuming new leafy foods.

Sugars

In the two grown-ups and kids, the admission of free sugars ought to be diminished to under 10% of absolute energy consumption (2, 7). A decrease to under 5% of complete energy admission would give extra medical advantages (7).

Consuming free sugars expands the gamble of dental caries (tooth rot). Overabundance calories from food sources and savors high free sugars additionally add to undesirable weight gain, which can prompt overweight and stoutness. Ongoing proof likewise shows that free sugars impact circulatory strain and serum lipids, and recommends that a decrease in free sugars consumption lessens risk factors for cardiovascular illnesses (13).

<u>Sugars intake can be decreased by</u>:

- restricting the utilization of food varieties and beverages containing high measures of sugars, for example, sweet bites, confections and sugar-improved drinks (for example a wide range of refreshments containing free sugars - these incorporate carbonated or non-carbonated sodas, natural product or vegetable squeezes and beverages, fluid and powder concentrates, enhanced water, energy and sports drinks, ready-to-drink tea, ready-to-drink espresso and seasoned milk drinks); and
- eating new leafy foods vegetables as snacks rather than sweet tidbits.

advancing sound weight control plans

Diet develops over the long run, being impacted by numerous social and monetary elements that collaborate in a mind boggling way to shape individual dietary examples. These variables incorporate pay, food costs (which will influence the accessibility and reasonableness of quality food sources), individual inclinations and convictions, social practices, and topographical and natural angles (counting environmental change). In this manner, advancing a good food climate - including food frameworks that advance an enhanced, adjusted and solid eating regimen - requires the contribution of various areas and partners, including government, and the general population and confidential areas.

States play a focal part in establishing a good food climate that empowers individuals to embrace and keep up with sound dietary practices. Compelling activities by strategy creators to establish a quality food climate incorporate the accompanying:

- Making soundness in public strategies and money growth strategies - including exchange, food and rural approaches - to advance a solid eating regimen and safeguard general wellbeing through:

- expanding impetuses for makers and retailers to develop, use and sell new foods grown from the ground;
- lessening impetuses for the food business to proceed or build creation of handled food varieties containing elevated degrees of soaked fats, trans-fats, free sugars and salt/sodium;
- empowering reformulation of food items to diminish the items in immersed fats, trans-fats, free sugars and salt/sodium, determined to kill mechanically delivered trans-fats;
- laying out principles to encourage sound dietary practices through guaranteeing the accessibility of solid, nutritious, protected and reasonable food sources in pre-schools, schools, other public establishments and the work environment;
- investigating administrative and intentional instruments (for example promoting guidelines and sustenance marking strategies), and financial motivating forces or disincentives (for example tax collection and endowments) to advance a solid eating regimen; and

- empowering transnational, public and neighborhood food administrations and catering outlets to work on the nourishing nature of their food varieties - guaranteeing the accessibility and moderateness of solid decisions - and survey segment sizes and valuing.

Empowering customer interest for quality food sources and dinners through:

- advancing buyer consciousness of a sound eating routine;
- creating school strategies and projects that urge youngsters to embrace and keep a sound eating routine;
- teaching kids, teenagers and grown-ups about sustenance and solid dietary practices;
- empowering culinary abilities, remembering for kids through schools;
- supporting retail location data, including through nourishment naming that guarantees precise, normalized and conceivable data on supplement contents in food varieties (in accordance with the Codex Alimentarius Commission rules), with the

expansion of front-of-pack marking to work with buyer understanding; and

- giving nourishment and dietary advising at essential medical services offices.

Advancing suitable baby and small kid taking care of practices through:

- Carrying out the Global Code of Advertising of Bosom milk Substitutes and resulting applicable World Wellbeing Get together goals;
- Carrying out arrangements and practices to advance security of working moms; and
- Advancing, securing and supporting breastfeeding in wellbeing administrations and the local area, including through the Child amicable Clinic Drive.

Chapter 2

Consume less salt and sugar

Filipinos consume two times the suggested measure of sodium, jeopardizing them of hypertension, which thusly builds the gamble of coronary illness and stroke. The vast majority help their sodium through salt. Diminish your salt admission to 5g each day, comparable to around one teaspoon. It's more straightforward to do this by restricting how much salt, soy sauce, fish sauce and other high-sodium fixings while getting ready dinners; eliminating salt, flavors and sauces from your feast table; staying away from pungent bites; and picking low-sodium items.

Then again, consuming inordinate measures of sugars expands the gamble of tooth rot and unfortunate weight gain. In the two grown-ups and youngsters, the admission of free sugars ought to be diminished to under 10% of absolute energy consumption. This is identical to 50g or around 12 teaspoons for a grown-up. WHO suggests consuming under 5% of all out energy consumption for extra medical advantages. You can decrease your sugar admission by restricting the utilization of sweet tidbits, confections and sugar-improved refreshments.

Eat a solid eating routine all through your life to assist with forestalling all types of unhealthiness (squandering, hindering, underweight, insufficient nutrients or minerals, overweight, corpulence), as well as a scope of diet-related non-transmittable sicknesses (like coronary illness, stroke, diabetes and a few tumors), and lower your gamble of irresistible infections. Be that as it may, the expanded utilization of handled food, fast urbanization and changing ways of life have prompted a change in dietary examples. Individuals are currently devouring more food varieties high in energy, fats and free sugars or salt/sodium, and many don't eat sufficient fiber-rich natural products, vegetables and entire grains.

So to be better with a more grounded insusceptible framework, you ought to eat - delivered trans fats, limit day to day salt admission to under 5 grams each day and breaking point admission of free or added sugars.

Limit fat admission

Diminish sufficient fiber-rich natural products, vegetables and entire grains, limit fat utilization away from immersed fats to unsaturated fats, kill economically how much absolute fat admission to under 30% of complete energy admission to assist with forestalling unfortunate weight gain. Bring down your gamble of creating non-transferable illnesses (like coronary illness, stroke, diabetes and a few malignant growths) by: diminishing soaked fats (found in greasy meat, spread, coconut oil, cream, cheddar, ghee and fat) to under 10% of all out energy consumption; decreasing all out trans fats (tracked down in handled food, cheap food, nibble food, broiled food, frozen pizza, pies, treats, margarines and spreads) to under 1% of complete energy admission; and supplanting both with unsaturated fats (found in fish, avocado, nuts, olive oil, soy, canola, sunflower and corn oils).

You can lessen fat consumption by:

- Changing how you cook - eliminate the greasy piece of meat, utilize vegetable oil (not creature oil), and bubble, steam or heat as opposed to broil
- Staying away from handled food sources containing trans fats
- Restricting the utilization of food sources containing high measures of immersed fats.

Limit salt consumption

Decrease your salt utilization to the suggested degree of under 5 g each day. The vast majority consume an excess of sodium through salt (relating to a normal of 9-12 g of salt each day) and insufficient potassium. High salt utilization and deficient potassium consumption (under 3.5 g) add to hypertension, which thus expands the gamble of coronary illness and stroke.

Individuals are frequently ignorant about how much salt they consume. In numerous nations, most salt comes from handled food sources (for example prepared feasts; handled meats like bacon, ham and salami; cheddar and pungent tidbits) or from food devoured often in enormous sums (for example bread). Salt is likewise added to food during preparing (for example bouillon, stock shapes, soy sauce and fish sauce) or at the table (for example table salt).

You can diminish salt utilization by:

- Not adding salt, soy sauce or fish sauce during the readiness of food
- Not having salt on the table
- Restricting the utilization of pungent tidbits
- Checking food marks and picking items with lower sodium content
- Consuming new foods grown from the ground to increment potassium, which can moderate the

adverse consequences of raised sodium utilization on circulatory strain.

Limit sugar consumption

Decrease your admission of free sugars all through the existence course. Free sugars are sugars added to food sources or beverages (for example glucose, galactose, fructose, sucrose or table sugar) by the producer, cook or customer, as well as sugars normally present in honey, syrups, natural product squeezes and organic product juice condensed.

Grown-ups and kids: diminish admission of free sugars to under 10% of complete energy consumption. A decrease to under 5% of all out energy consumption gives extra medical advantages, so diminish admission of free sugars further. Consuming free sugars expands the gamble of dental caries (tooth rot). Abundance calories from food sources and savors high free sugars additionally add to unfortunate weight gain, which can prompt overweight and stoutness.

<u>You can decrease your sugar admission by</u>:

- Restricting the utilization of food sources and beverages containing high measures of sugars (for example sugar-improved refreshments, sweet bites and confections)
- Eating new foods grown from the ground vegetables as snacks rather than sweet bites.

Chapter 3

Lessen consumption of harmful fats

Fats consumed ought to be under 30% of your complete energy consumption. This will assist with forestalling unfortunate weight gain and NCDs. There are various sorts of fats, yet unsaturated fats are best over soaked fats and trans-fats. WHO prescribes diminishing soaked fats to under 10% of complete energy admission; decreasing trans-fats to under 1% of all out energy admission; and supplanting both immersed fats and trans-fats to unsaturated fats.

The ideal unsaturated fats are tracked down in fish, avocado and nuts, and in sunflower, soybean, canola and olive oils; immersed fats are found in greasy meat, margarine, palm and coconut oil, cream, cheddar, ghee and fat; and trans-fats are tracked down in heated and broiled food sources, and pre-bundled bites and food sources, like frozen pizza, treats, bread rolls, and cooking oils and spreads.

Immersed fat is seen as in:

- spread, ghee, suet, fat, coconut oil and palm oil
- cakes
- bread rolls
- greasy cuts of meat
- wieners
- bacon
- relieved meats like salami, chorizo and pancetta
- cheddar
- baked goods, for example, pies, quiches, frankfurter rolls and croissants
- cream, crème fraîche and sharp cream
- frozen yogurt
- coconut milk and coconut cream
- milkshakes
- chocolate and chocolate spreads

Wellbeing rules suggest that :

- the typical man matured 19 to 64 years ought to eat something like 30g of soaked fat a day
- the typical lady matured 19 to 64 years ought to eat something like 20g of soaked fat a day

It's likewise suggested that individuals ought to diminish their general fat admission and supplant soaked fat with some unsaturated fat, including omega-3 fats.

Eating less fat

To assist you with cutting the aggregate sum of fat in your eating regimen:

- analyze food marks when you shop so you can pick food sources that are lower in fat
- barbecue, prepare, poach or steam food as opposed to broiling or cooking
- measure oil with a teaspoon to control the sum you use, or utilize an oil splash
- cut back noticeable excess and take the skin off meat and poultry prior to cooking it
- pick more streamlined cuts of meat that are lower in fat, for example, turkey bosom and diminished fat mince
- make your meat stews and curries go further by adding vegetables and beans
- attempt diminished fat spreads, for example, spreads in light of olive or sunflower oils

Eliminating soaked fat

<u>Commonsense tips to assist you with explicitly eliminating immersed fat</u>:

At the shops

Sustenance names on the front and back of bundling can assist you with eliminating immersed fat. Pay special attention to "soaks" or "sat fat" on the name.

High: More than 5g immerses per 100g. Might be variety coded red.

Medium: Somewhere in the range of 1.5g and 5g soaks per 100g. Might be variety coded golden.

Low: 1.5g immerses or less per 100g. Might be variety coded green.

This is an illustration of a name that shows a thing is high in soaked fat on the grounds that the immerses segment is variety coded red.

Expect to pick items with green or golden for soaked fat. There can be a major distinction in immersed fat substance between comparable items.

Pick the food that is lower in immersed fat. Serving sizes can shift as well, so ensure you're contrasting like for like. The most straightforward method for doing this is by taking a gander at the healthful substance per 100g.

At home

Spaghetti bolognese: utilize a lower-fat mince, as it's lower in immersed fat. In the event that you are not utilizing lower-fat mince, brown the mince first, then channel off the fat prior to adding different fixings. On the other hand, blend meat mince with a without meat mince elective.

Pizza: pick a lower-fat fixing, for example, vegetables, chicken, fish and other fish rather than additional cheddar or restored meats like pepperoni, salami and bacon.

Fish pie: utilize diminished fat spread and 1% fat milk to decrease the fat in the pound and sauce.

Stew: use lower-fat mince or blend in a sans meat mince elective. Or on the other hand, make a vegan stew utilizing blended beans, a few lentils and vegetables. Beans and lentils can combine with your 5 Per Day, as well.

Chips: pick thick, straight-cut chips rather than french fries or crease slice to lessen the surface region presented to fat. On the off chance that you're making your own, cook them in the stove with just enough Sunflower oil and the skins on, as opposed to profound broiling.

Potatoes: make your dish potatoes better by cutting them into bigger parts than expected and utilizing only a bit of sunflower or olive oil.

Mashes potato: utilize diminished fat spread rather than margarine, and 1% fat milk or skimmed milk rather than entire or semi-skimmed milk.

Chicken: go for less fatty cuts, like chicken bosom. Before you eat it, take the skin off to diminish the immersed fat substance.

Bacon: pick back bacon rather than dirty bacon, which contains more fat. Barbecue as opposed to searing.

Eggs: get ready eggs without oil or spread. Poach, bubble or dry fry your eggs.

Pasta: attempt a tomato-put together sauce with respect to your pasta. It's lower in immersed fat than a rich or messy sauce.

Milk: utilize 1% fat milk on your cereal and in hot beverages. It has about around 50% of the immersed fat of semi-skimmed.

Cheddar: while utilizing cheddar to enhance a dish or sauce, attempt serious areas of strength for a cheddar, like diminished fat mature cheddar, as you'll require less. Make cheddar go further by grinding as opposed to cutting it.

Yogurt: pick a lower-fat and lower-sugar yogurt. There can be a major distinction between various items.

Eating out

<u>Tips to assist you with eliminating soaked fat while eating out.</u>

Espresso: trade huge entire milk espresso for ordinary "thin" ones. Try not to include cream top.

Curry: go for dry or tomato-based dishes, for example, roasted or madras, rather than velvety curries like korma, pasanda or masala. Pick plain rice and chapatti rather than pilau rice and naan.

Kebabs: go for a shish kebab with pitta bread and salad as opposed to a doner kebab.

Chinese: pick a lower-fat dish, for example, steamed fish, chicken slash suey or szechuan prawns.

Thai: attempt a sautéed or steamed dish containing chicken, fish or vegetables. Keep an eye out for curries that contain coconut milk, which is high in immersed fat. Assuming you pick one of these, make an effort not to eat all the sauce.

Nibble time: trade food varieties high in sugar, salt and fat, like chocolate, doughnuts and cakes, for:

- Some organic product
- Wholegrain toast
- Low-fat and lower-sugar yogurt
- A little small bunch of unsalted nuts
- A currant bun
- A cut of organic product portion

- A cut of malt portion

Chapter 4

Keep away from unsafe utilization of liquor

There is no protected level for drinking liquor, Polishing off liquor can prompt medical conditions like mental and social problems, including liquor reliance, major NCDs like liver cirrhosis, a few malignant growths and heart sicknesses, as well as wounds coming about because of brutality and street conflicts and crashes.

Liquor is a psychoactive substance with reliance creating properties that has been generally utilized in many societies for quite a long time. The destructive utilization of liquor causes a high weight of illness and has critical social and monetary results.

The destructive utilization of liquor can likewise bring about mischief to others, like relatives, companions, colleagues and outsiders.

Liquor utilization is a causal consider in excess of 200 illnesses, wounds and other ailments. Drinking liquor is related with a gamble of creating medical conditions like mental and social problems, including liquor reliance, and major non-transferable sicknesses like liver cirrhosis, a few tumors and cardiovascular infections.

A huge extent of the illness trouble owing to liquor utilization emerges from unexpected and deliberate wounds, including those because of street car accidents, savagery, and self destruction. Lethal liquor related wounds will quite often happen in somewhat more youthful age gatherings.

A causal relationship has been laid out between destructive drinking and frequency or results of irresistible sicknesses like tuberculosis and HIV/Helps.

Liquor utilization by a hopeful mother might cause fetal liquor disorder (FAS) and pre-term birth intricacies.

Factors influencing liquor utilization and liquor related harm

Different elements which influence the levels and examples of liquor utilization and the greatness of liquor related issues in populaces have been distinguished at individual and cultural levels.

Cultural elements incorporate degree of monetary turn of events, culture, normal practices, accessibility of liquor, and execution and requirement of liquor arrangements. Unfavorable wellbeing effects and social damage from a given level and example of drinking are more noteworthy for less fortunate social orders.

Individual elements incorporate age, orientation, family conditions and financial status. In spite of the fact that there is no single gamble factor that is prevailing, the more weaknesses an individual has, the more probable the individual is to foster liquor related issues because of liquor utilization. Less fortunate people experience more noteworthy wellbeing and social damages from liquor utilization than additional well-to-do people.

The effect of liquor utilization on constant and intense wellbeing results not entirely set in stone by the all out volume of liquor drank and the example of drinking, especially those examples which are related with episodes of weighty drinking.

The setting of drinking assumes a significant part in the event of liquor related hurt, especially because of liquor inebriation. Liquor utilization can have an effect not just on the rate of illnesses, wounds and other ailments, yet in addition on their results and how these develop over the long haul.

There are distinctions in sexual orientation in liquor related mortality and bleakness, as well as levels and examples of liquor utilization. The level of liquor inferable passings among men adds up to 7.7 % of all worldwide passings contrasted with 2.6 % of all passings among ladies. Complete liquor per capita utilization in 2016 among male and female consumers overall was on normal 19.4 liters of unadulterated liquor for guys and 7.0 liters for females.

Lessening the burden from destructive utilization of liquor

Wellbeing, security and financial issues owing to liquor can be diminished when state run administrations plan and carry out fitting arrangements.

Strategy producers are urged to make a move on systems that have demonstrated to be viable and savvy. These incorporate

- managing the showcasing of cocktails (specifically to more youthful individuals);
- managing and limiting the accessibility of liquor;
- instituting suitable beverage driving strategies;
- lessening interest through tax collection and evaluating instruments;
- bringing issues to light of the wellbeing and social issues for people and society at large caused by the unsafe utilization of liquor;
- guaranteeing support for viable liquor approaches;
- giving open and reasonable treatment to individuals with liquor use issues; and
- carrying out evaluating and brief mediation programs in wellbeing administrations for dangerous and destructive drinking.

Chapter 5

Be active

Active work is characterized as any substantial development delivered by skeletal muscles that requires energy consumption. This incorporates exercise and exercises embraced while working, playing, completing family errands, voyaging, and participating in sporting pursuits. How much actual work you want relies upon your age bunch yet grown-ups matured 18-64 years ought to do no less than 150 minutes of moderate-force physical

Good reasons to be more active

Innovation and things that assist us with going about our responsibilities or tasks quicker have made our lives a lot simpler. In any case, individuals sit much really during the day; for instance, driving, dealing with a PC, or staring at the television. In 2013 to 2014 somewhat over portion of Canadians, matured 12 years and more established, said they were decently dynamic in their relaxation time. This is an issue. Many individuals aren't adequately moving to remain sound.

Customary active work brings down your gamble of:

- hypertension, stroke, and coronary illness
- type 2 diabetes
- osteoporosis
- colon malignant growth
- heftiness
- tension
- gloom

Being active will likewise:

- give you more energy
- work on your stance and equilibrium
- assist you with remaining at a solid weight
- assist with helping you have an improved outlook on yourself

Being active Doesn't Need to Be Hard

The vast majority who dance, swim, play tennis, or go climbing do these exercises since they appreciate them. Having a great time is great for your wellbeing. Participating in an action that you appreciate will help you unwind and assist with bringing down your pressure. It will assist you with having a decent outlook on yourself, which is great for your psychological wellness.

What action requests to you? Attempt to find a movement you appreciate doing without help from anyone else or with others. Assuming that you like what you're doing you'll presumably continue to make it happen. Learn about exercises locally to attempt new things and acquire new abilities.

Active work doesn't need to be difficult to be really great for your body. In the event that you could do without going to a rec center, accomplish something outside or stroll in a shopping center.

Be active with Family and Make New Companions

Your time is quite possibly of the most valuable gift you can give your loved ones. Invest more energy outside with your accomplice and youngsters. Walk the canine, play at a recreation area, or show your kids a game from your young life. These are ways of appreciating natural air and open space of the outside. In the event that the weather conditions isn't great, contemplate taking your youngsters and their grandparents to a historical center. Stroll through the presentations and pay attention to their accounts from an earlier time.

Getting dynamic can be an opportunity to make new companions. Bunch exercises at a local area or sporting (rec) focus can give you social help and a spot to feel like you have a place. Look at programs in your space and converse with your companions about exercises that they do.

Remain active so You'll be Free as You Age

Active work can assist you with living better as you become older. Remaining dynamic will assist you with coming to, twist, lift, convey, and move around more straightforward, so you can continue to do things you like to do. The more you sit or lie around, the stiffer your joints get. Extending and strength activities will keep your muscles and joints moving and assist with halting falls and wounds.

Being dynamic is ok for a great many people. Begin gradually and move gradually up. On the off chance that you can't say much about how much action you can do, converse with your medical care supplier.

Active work needn't bother with to be dull or exhausting. Do exercises you appreciate more regularly. You wouldn't believe how rapidly you begin to feel more grounded and like you have more energy.

The significance of being actually active outside

Searching for a method for getting solid? Go outside for a walk or a bicycle ride. Strolling or being truly dynamic outside is a simple, minimal expense method for helping your psychological well-being. It can further develop your wellness level and you get other medical advantages as well.

Youngsters

Being truly dynamic outside can help your body, psyche, and soul. Assuming your youngster is dynamic outside on a more regular basis, it can assist with bringing down the gamble of medical conditions like weight. It can likewise:

- decline side effects of consideration shortfall and hyperactivity issue (ADHD)
- increment vitamin D, which might assist with forestalling bone issues, coronary illness, and diabetes
- assists them with seeing distances better and brings down the gamble of astigmatism

Being outside more frequently can assist your youngster with getting to realize their local better. This can cause them to be more self-assured.

Grown-ups

Investing more energy being dynamic outside can assist you with dealing with your weight better. It might likewise give you other medical advantages like:

- supporting your emotional wellness
- expanding energy
- bringing down your gamble of diabetes, coronary illness, and a few kinds of disease

Being outside more can likewise help you have a positive outlook on and need to engage locally.

Grown-ups and youngsters can profit from being dynamic outside and investing energy with loved ones. Numerous recollections are made when individuals invest energy outside together.

Chapter 6

Check your blood pressure consistently

Hypertension, or hypertension, is known as a "quiet executioner". This is on the grounds that many individuals who have hypertension may not know about the issue as it might not have any side effects. Whenever left uncontrolled, hypertension can prompt heart, cerebrum, kidney and different infections. Have your pulse really looked at consistently by a wellbeing laborer so you know your numbers. On the off chance that your pulse is high, get the guidance of a wellbeing specialist. This is crucial in the avoidance and control of hypertension.

Checking circulatory strain at home is a significant piece of overseeing hypertension (hypertension).

The American Heart Affiliation (AHA) and different associations suggest that individuals with hypertension screen their pulse at home. Consistently checking pulse at home assists your consideration suppliers with deciding whether treatment is working.

Home circulatory strain screens are accessible generally and without a solution. In any case, it means quite a bit to know how to find a decent home circulatory strain screen and to accurately utilize it.

requirements to screen circulatory strain at home

Observing your pulse at home can:

- Assist with early analysis. Self-observing can assist your wellbeing with caring supplier analyze hypertension sooner than if you have just periodic pulse readings in a clinical office. Home checking is particularly significant for individuals with raised circulatory strain or another condition that could add to hypertension, like diabetes or kidney issues.
- Assist with following your treatment. The best way to know whether your way of life changes or meds are working is to check your circulatory

strain routinely. Observing pulse changes at home can assist you and your consideration supplier with coming to conclusions about treatment, for example, changing measurements or evolving drugs.

- Energize better control. Self-observing can provide you with a more grounded feeling of command over your wellbeing. Self-observing could assist you with feeling more persuaded to control your pulse with further developed diet, active work and legitimate prescription use.

- Reduce your medical care expenses. Self-checking could assist with eliminating clinical visits.

- Check in the event that your circulatory strain varies outside a clinical office. Certain individuals have spikes in circulatory strain because of apprehension during a clinical visit (white coat hypertension). Others whose pulse is alright at a facility have worse hypertension somewhere else (veiled hypertension). Checking circulatory strain at home can help decide whether you have genuine hypertension.

Not every person can follow circulatory strain at home. For those with unpredictable pulses, home circulatory strain screens probably won't give an exact perusing.

Kinds of home screens

Most drug stores, clinical stock stores and a few sites sell home pulse screens. Specialists suggest a programmed or electronic gadget. Your medical care supplier can assist you with picking the screen that is best for you.

Pulse screens by and large have similar fundamental parts:

- Inflatable sleeve. The sleeve's inward layer loads up with air and presses the arm. The sleeve's external layer has a clasp to hold the sleeve set up. The gadget computes pulse and blood stream by estimating the progressions in the movement of the vein as the blood courses through while the sleeve collapses.
- Measure for readouts. Some pulse screens can take a few readings and report the midpoints.

Advanced screens that are fitted on the upper arm are by and large the most reliable.

Certain individuals with extremely enormous arms might not approach a well-fitting upper arm sleeve at home. Assuming this is the case, estimating circulatory strain at the wrist or lower arm might be alright whenever utilized as coordinated and checked against estimations taken in your supplier's office. For the most solid circulatory strain estimation, the American Heart Affiliation suggests utilizing a screen with a sleeve that circumvents your upper arm, when accessible.

For individuals who can't check pulse at home, numerous drug stores and stores have public circulatory strain gadgets. The exactness of these gadgets might change.

Elements to consider

While picking a pulse screen, consider:

- Sleeve size. It is critical to Have an appropriately fitting sleeve. Sleeves that fit inadequately won't give exact pulse estimations. Ask your medical care supplier what sleeve size you want.

- Show. The presentation that shows pulse estimations ought to be clear and simple to peruse.
- Cost. Costs shift. Inquire as to whether your strategy takes care of the expense of a home circulatory strain screen.

Gadget precision

One time each year, check the exactness of your screen by carrying it to your supplier's office and contrasting your screen's readings and those taken at the workplace.

Tips for precise use

Regardless of what sort of home pulse screen you pick, legitimate use requires preparing and practice. Take the gadget to your medical care supplier to ensure the one you've picked is the best fit for you. Figure out how to accurately utilize the screen.

To assist with guaranteeing precise circulatory strain checking at home:

- Check to be certain your gadget is right. Prior to utilizing a screen, have your medical services supplier contrast the readings from your screen and the readings from the screen in the clinical office. Additionally have your supplier watch you utilize the gadget to check whether you're doing it appropriately. Assuming you drop the gadget or harm it, have it checked prior to utilizing it once more.

- Toward the start, measure your circulatory strain no less than two times day to day. Take it first toward the beginning of the prior day eating or taking any prescriptions. Take it again at night. Each time you measure, take a few readings to ensure your outcomes are something similar. Your medical services supplier could suggest taking your circulatory strain at similar times every day.

- Try not to quantify your circulatory strain just after you awaken. You can plan for the afternoon, however don't have breakfast or take drugs prior to estimating your pulse. On the off chance that you practice subsequent to waking, take your pulse prior to working out.

- Stay away from food, caffeine, tobacco and liquor for 30 minutes prior to taking a perusing. Likewise, void your bladder first. A full bladder can increment circulatory strain somewhat.
- Sit unobtrusively previously and during checking. At the point when you're prepared to take your circulatory strain, sit for five minutes in an agreeable situation with your legs and lower legs uncrossed. Your back ought to be upheld against a seat. Attempt to be quiet and not contemplate upsetting things. Try not to talk while taking your circulatory strain.
- Ensure your arm is situated appropriately. Continuously utilize a similar arm while taking your pulse. Rest your arm, raised to the level of your heart, on a table, work area or seat arm. You could have to put a pad or pad under your arm to raise it sufficiently high.

- Put the sleeve on uncovered skin, not over apparel. A rolled-up sleeve that is tight around your arm can influence the perusing. You might have to slip your arm out of the sleeve.
- Take a recurrent perusing. Stand by 1 to 3 minutes after the principal perusing, and afterward take another. In the event that your screen doesn't monitor pulse readings or pulses, get them on paper.

Pulse fluctuates over the course of the day. Readings are in many cases a little higher in the first part of the day. Likewise, your pulse may be marginally lower at home than in a clinical office.

Contact your medical care supplier on the off chance that you have any strange expansions in your pulse or on the other hand assuming your circulatory strain stays higher than expected. Ask your supplier at what perusing you ought to summon the clinical office right.

Following your circulatory strain readings

Certain individuals utilize a note pad to record their circulatory strain readings.

In the event that you have an electronic individual wellbeing record, you could decide to record your data utilizing a PC or cell phone. This provides you with the choice of imparting your readings to your medical care suppliers and relatives. Some circulatory strain screens transfer this information naturally.

Long-term benefits

Assuming that your pulse is very much controlled, ask your medical care supplier how frequently you want to actually look at it. You could possibly take a look at it just one time each day or on rare occasions. In the event that you're simply beginning home observing or evolving treatment, your supplier could suggest checking pulse beginning fourteen days after treatment changes and seven days before your next arrangement.

Home pulse checking is definitely not a substitute for clinical visits. Home circulatory strain screens could not be right all of the time. Regardless of whether you get readings that are run of the mill for you, don't stop or change your prescriptions or your eating routine without conversing with your consideration supplier first. Be that as it may, assuming proceeded with home checking shows your pulse is taken care of, you could possibly make less clinical visits.

Chapter 7

Practice safe sex

Taking care of your sexual wellbeing is significant for your general wellbeing and prosperity. Practice safe sex to forestall HIV and other physically communicated diseases like gonorrhea and syphilis. There are accessible avoidance measures, for example, pre-openness prophylaxis (PrEP) that will shield you from HIV and condoms that will safeguard you from HIV and other STIs.

Unprotected sex might jeopardize you of STIs

Perilous sex might endanger you or your sexual accomplices of STIs. This doesn't simply mean genital sex however any type of sexual contact (this incorporates butt-centric, oral, vaginal and a skin-to-skin contact).

Certain STIs (like syphilis and genital moles) can spread by engaging in sexual relations with a tainted accomplice when a sore or rash is available.

Unborn infants are additionally in danger as well, since some STIs like inherent syphilis and HIV, can pass from mother to child during pregnancy and upon entering the world.

Whenever left untreated, STIs can cause difficult ailment and affect your wellbeing (counting pelvic provocative sickness (PID) and fruitlessness in people.

STIs are normal. A few kinds of STIs include:

- chlamydia
- gonorrhea
- syphilis
- genital moles
- genital herpes
- HIV
- hepatitis A, B and C
- mycoplasma genitalium.

Not all STIs have clear side effects so you and your sexual accomplices may not know that you have a STI.

That is the reason rehearsing safe sex is significant. Use condoms for more secure sex.

Condoms (likewise called sheaths or rubbers) give the best security against STIs. They go about as an actual hindrance to forestall the trading of body liquids.

In spite of the fact that there is no assurance that condoms and other hindrance techniques give 100 percent security against STIs, they assist sex with being more secure when utilized accurately.

Sorts of condoms

Condoms are a type of obstruction contraception - fundamentally their responsibility is to prevent sperm from entering the vagina, mouth or rear-end and diminish our gamble of getting STIs.

Kinds of boundary strategies include:

- Male (or outer) condoms - a flimsy solid plastic (elastic) pocket that come in various sizes and styles. (Not one size fits all.) Non-plastic condoms are accessible for individuals who are hypersensitive to plastic.

- Female (or inward) condoms - a delicate pocket made of engineered elastic (seems to be an outside condom) with 2 adaptable rings at each end. These condoms come in one size and are as of now greased up, they are intended to fit inside the vagina or rear-end.

- stomach - a delicate, shallow cup made of silicone that fits inside the vagina and covers the cervix (access to the uterus or belly). Stomachs give great assurance against pregnancy, yet they don't shield you from STIs.

Condoms are accessible from stores, drug stores (or scientific experts), sexual wellbeing facilities and family arranging centers. They can likewise be bought from candy machines at certain clubs, bars, schools and colleges.

Having more secure sex with condoms and other hindrance techniques

Follow these basic hints while utilizing condoms and other hindrance strategies:

- Continuously utilize a new, greased up condom each time you engage in sexual relations.
- Really look at the utilization by date - don't utilize a condom past its expiry date.
- While opening the bundle, be mindful so as not to tear the condom with fingernails, gems or teeth.
- Assuming that you want additional oil, utilize just water-based ointments. Different greases can harm the condom.
- Condoms ought to be utilized from the outset of sex as far as possible. STIs can be sent when your accomplice pre-discharges ('pre-cums') on excitement.
- Use condoms on vibrators and sex toys you share with accomplices.
- Medical gloves can be worn during 'fingering' of the vagina or butt.
- Utilize dental dams (a sheet of plastic worn over the female privates) during oral sex.
- Recall that a stomach (a cap worn high in the vagina to cover the cervix) gives low security against STIs.

Instructions to utilize condoms effectively

Condoms, in any event, when utilized accurately, don't ensure 100 percent assurance against STIs or spontaneous pregnancy.

Remember that condoms:

- May break, particularly on the off chance that they are not put away as expected or a water-based oil isn't utilized.
- Try not to cover the whole genital skin region so you might in any case get a STI (like pubic lice, scabies, genital moles and genital herpes) through skin-to-skin contact.
- Work best with water-based ointment - oil-based grease will in general reason breakage.
- Can be harmed in heat - particularly on the off chance that they have been put away in hot spots, (for example, in vehicle glove boxes) for extensive stretches.
- Have an expiry date and can't be utilized past their utilization by date.
- Are for single utilize just and can't be reused.

Different tips for more secure sex

Sex ought to be charming. More secure sex implies sexual contact when you and your accomplice/s are prepared. Any type of sex should be consensual, and you ought to feel regarded and secured. This incorporates:

- Vaginal sex - embedding a penis into a vagina.
- Butt-centric sex - embedding your penis or different items, (for example, sex toys, dildos, fingers) into your accomplice's rear-end.
- Oral sex - utilizing your mouth, lips or tongue to animate your accomplice's private parts or butt.

Ways that you can rehearse more secure sex include:

- Chat with your accomplice transparently about your sexual wellbeing. Convey your sexual necessities and what you need to physically investigate.
- Limit your number of sexual accomplices.
- Get tried for STIs.

- In the event that you have a STI, get treated. Stay away from sexual contact until you get clinical exhortation that you are presently not irresistible.

- In the event that somebody is constraining you to have intercourse or causes you to feel awkward, tell them. By regulation, sex should be consensual, which likewise implies regarding others' choices when they say 'no' or on the other hand assuming they are excessively out of it to assent.

- Keep away from sex on the off chance that you are impacted by medications and liquor. It can cloud your judgment and you could do things you later lament.

- Utilize different kinds of contraception notwithstanding a condom to try not to get pregnant.

It's really smart to keep away from sex if your sexual accomplice/s:

- Has wounds, cuts, ulcers, rankles, moles or rashes around their privates, mouth or butt (like hemorrhoids and butt-centric gaps)
- Has unhealed or excited piercings in their mouth or privates
- Has a throat disease
- Is a lady and has her period.

Other more secure sexual practices

- Since you have more secure sex, doesn't mean it must drag. Keep in mind, making closeness in a relationship takes time.
- Having intercourse is just a single piece of sexual closeness and there are alternate ways of acquiring sexual delight including foreplay and actual contact.

A few different types of sexual lead that can lessen your gamble of STIs include:

Kissing, Snuggling, Back rub, Masturbation (independently or with sexual accomplices) discharging on whole skin, Sex utilizing hindrance contraception - like a condoms.

Keep in mind, it's smarter to stay away from sexual contact in the event that you or your accomplice have any wounds, rashes or ulcers.

Keeping away from dangerous circumstances

A few circumstances can expand your gamble of risky sex. It's smarter to stay away from circumstances where you can lessen your gamble of getting a STI. These include:

- Being intoxicated or out of it on medications can prompt impeded independent direction
- Feeling compelled to have intercourse
- Feeling that it's alright 'one time only'
- Accepting you can perceive somebody has a STI in light of the fact that they will have side effects.
- In the event that you feel awkward in any circumstance, it's OK to say no.

Conquering boundaries to safe sex

Keep in mind, rehearsing safe sex doesn't need to be a drag and is delighted in by bunches of individuals. In the event that you are finding it hard to tell how to begin, you might discover a portion of these ideas valuable:

- Be ready. Continuously convey condoms with you and keep them helpful at home, so you don't need to hinder engaging in sexual relations to search for one.
- Assuming you find condoms decrease your sexual joy, put some water-put together grease with respect to the tip for additional inclination and responsiveness.
- Figure out how to utilize condoms. They might take a little becoming acclimated to, yet it's superior to getting a STI.
- Include condoms in foreplay.
- On the off chance that you are awkward purchasing condoms over the counter in shops, they are accessible from candy machines, on the web or from local area wellbeing or sexual wellbeing facilities.

- Hormonal contraception like the pill, little pill, vaginal ring and long-acting converse contraception or LARC (counting inserts, IUDs, infusions) just give assurance against spontaneous pregnancy and not against STIs.
- Focus on your sexual wellbeing - it is significant. Instruct yourself about STIs. Anybody who has intercourse or engages in sexual relations in the past is in danger.
- Try not to figure you can determine whether somebody has a STI by simply checking them out. Numerous STIs have no undeniable signs.
- Be careful that STIs are normal - they don't imply that you are 'filthy' or 'modest'.
- Get tried for STIs in the event that you are physically dynamic, particularly assuming you engage in sexual relations without a condom. All accomplices ought to be tried.

What to do on the off chance that you suspect a few side effects of STI

STIs are normal and the vast majority will get a STI in the course of their life. Most STIs are reparable, and all can be dealt with. The best exhortation on the off chance that you are physically dynamic is to get tried consistently - no less than one time each year.

Get tried all the more regularly on the off chance that you:

- are a gay man or a man who has intercourse with different men - something like once consistently
- have numerous sexual accomplices over a brief period (for instance, in excess of 10 accomplices in 90 days) - like clockwork.

Typically, a basic blood or pee test is everything necessary.

It's vital to get tried if:

- you notice side effects in the wake of engaging in sexual relations without a condom
- the condom broke or slipped during sex
- you start another relationship (counting relaxed accomplices)

- you are anticipating beginning a family, or you are pregnant.

Assuming you figure you might have or have been presented to a STI, proceed to chat with your nearby specialist, medical caretaker or wellbeing laborer, who can assist you with getting the tests you want to reassure you. Testing, and treatment where essential, along with condoms, remove the concern from sex.

Chapter 8

Converse with somebody you trust assuming you're feeling down

Despondency is a typical sickness overall with more than 260 million individuals impacted. Despondency can appear in changed ways, yet it could cause you to feel irredeemable or useless, or you could ponder negative and upsetting considerations a ton or have a mind-boggling feeling of agony. Assuming you're going through this, recall that you are in good company. Converse with somebody you trust, for example, a relative, companion, partner or emotional well-being proficient about how you feel.

Sadness is a typical sickness around the world, with an expected 3.8% of the populace impacted, including 5.0% among grown-ups and 5.7% among grown-ups more established than 60 years (1). Roughly 280 million individuals on the planet have sadness (1). Sadness is unique in relation to regular temperament vacillations and brief profound reactions to challenges in daily existence. Particularly when intermittent and with moderate or extreme force, wretchedness might turn into a serious medical issue. It can make the impacted individual endure significantly and capability ineffectively working, at school and in the family. Even from a pessimistic standpoint, sadness can prompt self destruction. More than 700 ,000 individuals bite the dust because of self destruction consistently. Self destruction is the fourth driving reason for death in 15-29-year-olds.

In spite of the fact that there are known, powerful medicines for mental problems, over 75% of individuals in low-and center pay nations get no treatment (2). Hindrances to powerful mind incorporate an absence of assets, absence of prepared medical services suppliers and social shame related with mental issues. In nations of all pay levels, individuals who experience discouragement are frequently not accurately analyzed, and other people who don't have the issue are again and again misdiagnosed and recommended antidepressants.

Side effects and examples

During a burdensome episode, the individual encounters discouraged temperament (feeling miserable, crabby, vacant) or a deficiency of joy or interest in exercises, for the vast majority of the day, essentially consistently, for something like fourteen days. A few different side effects are likewise present, which might incorporate unfortunate focus, sensations of extreme responsibility or low self-esteem, sadness about the future, contemplations about passing on or self destruction, upset rest, changes in hunger or weight, and feeling particularly drained or low in energy.

In a few social settings, certain individuals might communicate their temperament changes all the more promptly as substantial side effects (for example torment, exhaustion, shortcoming). However, these actual side effects are not because of another ailment.

During a burdensome episode, the individual encounters critical trouble in private, family, social, instructive, word related, or potentially other significant areas of working.

A burdensome episode can be sorted as gentle, moderate, or serious relying upon the number and seriousness of side effects, as well as the effect on the singular's working.

There are various examples of temperament problems including:

- single episode burdensome confusion, meaning the individual's sole episode);
- intermittent burdensome problem, meaning the individual has a past filled with no less than two burdensome episodes; and
- bipolar turmoil, implying that burdensome episodes substitute with times of hyper side effects, which incorporate elation or peevishness, expanded action or energy, and different side effects like expanded loquacity, dashing contemplations, expanded confidence, diminished need for rest, distractibility, and incautious foolish way of behaving.

Contributing variables and counteraction

Discouragement results from a complicated collaboration of social, mental, and natural elements. Individuals who have carried on with antagonistic life altering situations (joblessness, deprivation, horrible accidents) are bound to foster despondency. Misery can, thusly, lead to more pressure and brokenness and deteriorate the impacted individual's life circumstance and the actual downturn.

There are interrelationships among gloom and actual wellbeing. For instance, cardiovascular sickness can prompt discouragement as well as the other way around.

Anticipation programs have been displayed to diminish sadness. Successful people group ways to deal with forestall sadness incorporate school-based projects to improve an example of positive adapting in kids and teenagers. Intercessions for guardians of kids with social issues might lessen parental burdensome side effects and further develop results for their youngsters. Practice programs for more seasoned people can likewise be compelling in wretchedness counteraction.

Diagnosis and treatment

There are viable medicines for sorrow.

Contingent upon the seriousness and example of burdensome episodes over the long run, medical care suppliers might offer mental therapies like social enactment, mental conduct treatment and relational psychotherapy, as well as stimulant drug like specific serotonin reuptake inhibitors (SSRIs) and tricyclic antidepressants (TCAs). Various drugs are utilized for bipolar confusion. Medical care suppliers ought to remember the conceivable unfriendly impacts related with energizer medicine, the capacity to convey either mediation (regarding skill, or potentially therapy accessibility), and individual inclinations. Different mental treatment designs for thought incorporate individual and additionally bunch eye to eye mental medicines conveyed by experts and regulated lay specialists. Antidepressants are not the main line of treatment for gentle gloom. They ought not be utilized for treating discouragement in youngsters and are not the first line of treatment in quite a while, among whom they ought to be utilized with additional mindfulness.

Chapter 9

Drink safe water

Drinking risky water can prompt water-borne illnesses, for example, cholera, looseness of the bowels, hepatitis A, typhoid and polio. Universally, something like 2 billion individuals utilize a drinking water source polluted with dung. Check with your water concessionaire and water topping off station to guarantee that the water you're drinking is protected. In a setting where you are uncertain of your water source, heat up your water for something like one moment. This will obliterate unsafe creatures in the water. Allow it to cool normally prior to drinking.

Safe and promptly accessible water is significant for general wellbeing, whether it is utilized for drinking, homegrown use, food creation or sporting purposes. Further developed water supply and disinfection, and better administration of water assets, can support nations' financial development and can contribute enormously to neediness decrease.

Drinking-water administrations

Manageable Improvement objective 6.1 calls for widespread and evenhanded admittance to protected and reasonable drinking water. The objective is followed the mark of "securely oversaw drinking water administrations" - drinking water from a superior water source that is situated on premises, accessible when required, and free from waste and need synthetic tainting.

In 2020, 5.8 billion individuals utilized securely overseen drinking-water administrations - that is, they utilized better water sources situated on premises, accessible when required, and liberated from tainting. The excess 2 billion individuals without securely oversaw administrations in 2020 included:

- 1.2 billion individuals with essential administrations, meaning a superior water source situated inside a full circle of 30 minutes;
- 282 million individuals with restricted administrations, or a better water source requiring over 30 minutes to gather water;

- 368 million individuals taking water from unprotected wells and springs; and
- 122 million individuals gathering untreated surface water from lakes, lakes, streams and streams.

Sharp geographic, sociocultural and financial disparities continue, among rustic and metropolitan regions as well as in towns and urban areas where individuals residing in low-pay, casual or unlawful settlements normally have less admittance to further developed wellsprings of drinking-water than different occupants.

Water and wellbeing

Tainted water and unfortunate sterilization are connected to transmission of illnesses, for example, cholera, loose bowels, diarrhea, hepatitis A, typhoid and polio. Missing, insufficient, or improperly oversaw water and sterilization administrations open people to preventable wellbeing gambles. This is especially the situation in medical care offices where the two patients and staff are put at extra gamble of contamination and illness when water, sterilization and cleanliness administrations are deficient. Worldwide, 15% of patients foster a contamination during an emergency clinic stay, with the extent a lot more noteworthy in low-pay nations.

Deficient administration of metropolitan, modern and rural wastewater implies the drinking-water of a huge number of individuals is hazardously defiled or synthetically dirtied. Normal presence of synthetic substances, especially in groundwater, can likewise be of wellbeing importance, including arsenic and fluoride, while different synthetics, like lead, might be raised in drinking-water because of draining from water supply parts in touch with drinking-water.

Nearly 829 000 individuals are assessed to bite the dust every year from looseness of the bowels because of perilous drinking-water, sterilization and hand cleanliness. However the runs is generally preventable, and the passings of 297 000 kids matured under 5 years could be stayed away from every year in the event that these gamble factors were tended to. Where water isn't promptly accessible, individuals might choose handwashing isn't fundamentally important, subsequently adding to the probability of the runs and different infections.

Looseness of the bowels is the most commonly realized illness connected to sullied food and water however there are different perils. In 2017, more than 220 million individuals required deterrent therapy for schistosomiasis - an intense and ongoing sickness brought about by parasitic worms contracted through openness to pervaded water.

In many regions of the planet, bugs that live or raise in water convey and communicate illnesses like dengue fever. A portion of these bugs, known as vectors, breed in clean, as opposed to filthy water, and family drinking water holders can act as favorable places. The straightforward mediation of covering water capacity holders can diminish vector reproducing and may likewise lessen waste defilement of water at the family level.

Financial and social impacts

At the point when water comes from improved and more open sources, individuals invest less energy and exertion truly gathering it, meaning they can be useful in alternate ways. This can likewise bring about more prominent individual wellbeing and decreasing outer muscle issues by diminishing the need to make long or dangerous excursions to gather and convey water. Better water sources likewise mean less consumption on wellbeing, as individuals are more averse to become sick and bring about clinical expenses and are better ready to remain financially useful.

With kids especially in danger from water-related sicknesses, admittance to further developed wellsprings of water can bring about better wellbeing, and consequently better school participation, with positive longer-term ramifications for their lives.

Challenges

Authentic paces of progress would have to twofold for the world to accomplish all inclusive inclusion with essential drinking water administrations by 2030. To accomplish widespread securely overseen administrations, rates would have to fourfold. Environmental change, expanding water shortage, populace development, segment changes and urbanization as of now present difficulties for water supply frameworks. More than 2 billion individuals live in water-focused nations, as would be considered normal to be exacerbated in certain areas as consequence of environmental change and populace development. Re-utilization of wastewater to recuperate water, supplements or energy is turning into a significant methodology. Progressively nations are involving wastewater for water system; in non-industrial nations this addresses 7% of flooded land. While this training whenever done improperly presents wellbeing gambles, safe administration of wastewater can yield various advantages, including expanded food creation.

Choices for water sources utilized for drinking-water and water system will keep on developing, with a rising dependence on groundwater and elective sources, including wastewater. Environmental change will prompt more prominent vacillations in gathered water. The board of all water assets should be improved to guarantee arrangement and quality.

Chapter 10

Take anti-toxins just as recommended

Anti-infection obstruction is one of the greatest general wellbeing dangers in our age. At the point when antibiotics lose their power, bacterial contaminations become more enthusiastically to treat, prompting higher clinical expenses, delayed emergency clinic stays, and expanded mortality. Anti-infection agents are losing their power in view of abuse and abuse in people and creatures. Ensure you possibly take anti-toxins whenever recommended by a certified wellbeing proficient. Furthermore, when recommended, complete the treatment days as educated. Never share antibiotics.

Antibiotics are medications used to forestall and treat bacterial contaminations. Antibiotics opposition happens when microorganisms change in light of the utilization of these prescriptions.

Microorganisms, not people or creatures, become antibiotics safe. These microorganisms might taint people and creatures, and the diseases they cause are more enthusiastically to treat than those brought about by non-safe microbes.

Antibiotics opposition prompts higher clinical expenses, delayed medical clinic stays, and expanded mortality.

The world earnestly needs to have an impact on the manner in which it endorses and utilizes antibiotics. Regardless of whether new medications are created, without conduct change, anti-toxin obstruction will stay a significant danger. Conduct changes should likewise incorporate activities to lessen the spread of contaminations through immunization, hand washing, rehearsing more secure sex, and great food cleanliness.

Extent of the issue

Anti-toxin obstruction is ascending to perilously significant levels in all areas of the planet. New opposition components are arising and spreading around the world, compromising our capacity to treat normal irresistible infections. A developing rundown of contaminations -, for example, pneumonia, tuberculosis, blood harming, gonorrhea, and foodborne illnesses - are becoming more earnestly, and in some cases unthinkable, to treat as antibiotics become less compelling.

Where anti-infection agents can be purchased for human or creature use without a remedy, the development and spread of obstruction is exacerbated. Additionally, in nations without standard treatment rules, anti-infection agents are frequently over-endorsed by wellbeing laborers and veterinarians and over-utilized by the general population.

Without pressing activity, we are setting out toward a post-antibiotics period, where normal diseases and minor wounds can by and by kill.

Counteraction and control

Anti-toxin obstruction is advanced by the abuse and abuse of anti-toxins, as well as unfortunate contamination counteraction and control. Steps can be taken at all degrees of society to diminish the effect and breaking point the spread of obstruction.

People

To forestall and control the spread of anti-microbial obstruction, people can:

- Possibly use anti-infection agents when endorsed by a confirmed wellbeing proficient.
- Never request anti-toxins in the event that your wellbeing specialist says you don't require them.
- Continuously follow your wellbeing laborer's recommendation while utilizing antibiotics.
- Never offer or utilize extra antibiotics.
- Forestall contaminations by routinely washing hands, planning food cleanly, staying away from

close contact with wiped out individuals, rehearsing more secure sex, and staying up with the latest.

- Plan food cleanly, following the WHO Five Keys to More secure Food (keep perfect, separate crude and cooked, cook completely, guard food at temperatures, utilize safe water and unrefined substances) and pick food sources that have been created without the utilization of anti-toxins for development advancement or sickness counteraction in sound creatures.

Strategy producers

To forestall and control the spread of anti-infection opposition, strategy producers can:

- Guarantee a vigorous public activity intend to handle anti-infection obstruction is set up.
- Further develop reconnaissance of anti-toxin safe contaminations.
- Reinforce strategies, projects, and execution of disease avoidance and control measures.

- Direct and advance the proper use and removal of value prescriptions.
- Make data accessible on the effect of anti-infection obstruction.

Wellbeing experts

To forestall and control the spread of anti-microbial obstruction, wellbeing experts can:

- Forestall diseases by guaranteeing your hands, instruments, and climate are spotless.
- Possibly endorse and administer anti-toxins when they are required, as per current rules.
- Report anti-infection safe contaminations to reconnaissance groups.
- Converse with your patients about how to take anti-toxins accurately, anti-microbial opposition and the risks of abuse.
- Converse with your patients about forestalling diseases (for instance, inoculation, hand

washing, more secure sex, and covering nose and mouth while wheezing).

Medical services industry

To forestall and control the spread of anti-infection obstruction, the wellbeing business can:

- Put resources into innovative work of new anti-infection agents, immunizations, diagnostics and different apparatuses.

Agriculture area

To forestall and control the spread of anti-infection obstruction, the horticulture area can:

- Just give antibiotics to creatures under veterinary watch.
- Not use anti-infection agents for development advancement or to forestall sicknesses in sound creatures.
- Immunize creatures to diminish the requirement for anti-toxins and use options in contrast to antibiotics when accessible.

- Advance and apply great practices at all means of creation and handling of food sources from creature and plant sources.
- Further develop biosecurity on ranches and forestall diseases through superior cleanliness and animal government assistance.

Late turns of events

While there are a few new antibiotics being developed, not a solitary one of them are supposed to be powerful against the most hazardous types of anti-microbial safe microorganisms.

Given the simplicity and recurrence with which individuals currently travel, anti-infection opposition is a worldwide issue, requiring endeavors from all countries and numerous areas.

Influence

At the point when diseases can as of now not be treated by first-line anti-infection agents, more costly meds should be utilized. A more drawn out term of disease and treatment, frequently in clinics, increments medical care costs as well as the monetary weight on families and social orders.

Anti-infection opposition is endangering the accomplishments of present day medication. Organ transplantations, chemotherapy and medical procedures, for example, cesarean segments become substantially more risky without successful anti-infection agents for the counteraction and therapy of diseases.

About the Author

My name is Aileen R. Scott, am an American citizen, I work as a medical doctor and a marriage counsellor for 15 years , as a counsellor I help couples resolve conflict ,improve communication ,and strengthen their marriage and save a lot of marriages from destruction , 5 years ago I develop that passion of writing books, at first I took it as an hobby were I can write my feeling and thought ,but I get that idea on how to reach out to many people on how to save their marriage and how to live health on a daily basis through my books and thanks to amazon I can easily to that at the comfort of my home. My first book on amazon is "THE PERFECT LIFESTYLE OF MARRIAGE"

Am a single mother of two, am bless with two wonderful kids a boy and a girl, they mean the world to me.